Organizing with Feng Shui: 101 Tips Room by Room

by Bethany St. Clair

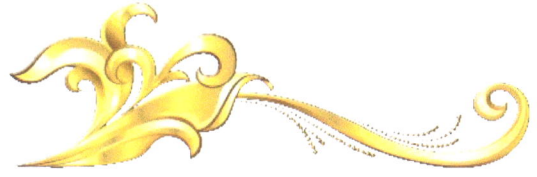

Organizing with Feng Shui: 101 Tips Room by Room
by Bethany St. Clair

Print: 978-0-9849546-0-5
Ebook: 978-09849546-4-3
Copyright © 2013, 2021 by Bethany St. Clair
All rights reserved. Except as permitted under
the U.S. Copyright Act of 1976

No part of this publication may be reproduced or transmitted in any form or by any means, electronic or mechanical, without permission from Bethany St. Clair.

Cover photo: Stas-Bejsov, iStockphoto.com

Published August 2013
First printing
Republished in 2022
Second printing

Dedicated to my Mother and all the ancestral women of my family who are healers.

Acknowledgements

A big thank you to Ralph Dranow, Erica Shelton, Damian Sol, Dr. Raphael Rettner, Anna Loi and Gerald F. Ward.

Introduction

Our physical space is a reflection of our inner space. Anywhere your space is cluttered, flow and harmony are impossible. This book provides basic tips to clear up your inner and outer space. Once your space is cleared, decision-making becomes easier, solutions present themselves, and the right people come into your life.

This book is a reminder if we've forgotten, or an entry point if we're unaware, to open up to healthy living and organized, functional work spaces. It is meant to be read in any order you choose. However, know that the most important rooms in your home are: the master bedroom, the kitchen, and the home office. Your intuition will guide you to go where you need to go.

When you begin the organizing process, drink plenty of water and stay well-hydrated. Begin in a small area of a room. There is a Japanese proverb that tells us: *you can't eat the apple in one bite, you must take small bites to finish the apple.* So start small, play your favorite music and work in one, or two hour blocks of time for the first few sessions until you have built up stamina for longer sessions. The only consideration I ask is that you finish one room, before going on to the next. If you feel overwhelmed, stop and rest for ten minutes. If you still feel overwhelmed, stop and put your things away and begin again the next day. If still overwhelmed, find a professional organizer, or ask a non-judgemental friend or relative to help. Always work in the daylight. The evening is time to rest and wind down. After your session, brush your hair and wash your hands up to the elbows to rid yourself of the sticky energy that has been built up. Continue to hydrate yourself for the next few days.

Here's to a fun, successful, beginning to welcoming new energy into your space.

"Your home should feel like a warm embrace every time you enter your space."
Bethany St. Clair

With Harmony and Love, Bethany

Table of Contents

Chapter 1: The Master Bedroom 1

Chapter 2: The Bathroom 3

Chapter 3: The Kitchen 5

Chapter 4: Children's Bedrooms 7

Chapter 5: The Media Room 9

Chapter 6: The Home Office/Your Work Space 11

Chapter 7: The Great Room 13

Chapter 8: The Garage 15

Chapter 9: The Entryway 18

Chapter 10: Closets 20

Bonus Feng Shui Tips 22

The Master Bedroom

The bedroom is where the harmony in the home begins and where sexual balance is restored. We spend one third of our lives sleeping, yet often the bedroom tends to be an afterthought or a dumping area for items that don't have a home. Ask yourself: does my bedroom look and feel warm, restful, and embracing?

Below are some tips for keeping this area in balance:

1. Avoid any clutter under the bed. The air should circulate from underneath the bed and around the room. If you have to have a platform bed with drawers for storage, it is best to keep soft items in the drawers; pillows, extra blankets, etc. Otherwise, purchase a bed with a bed frame.

2. If you have a television, computer, or workout equipment in the bedroom you are saying to the Universe that your relationship is with these items instead of your partner. Keep these items out of the bedroom even if you are single. Electronic equipment in the bedroom adds many electromagnetic fields that can zap us of energy. Research tells us high levels of electromagnetic fields (EMFs) weaken our immune system.

3. Have a solid headboard vs. one with iron bars or wrought iron. A solid wooden or upholstered headboard is best for grounding and sleeping through the night.

4. Place the location of your bed so you can see who is entering the bedroom from a sleeping position. In other words, you should be looking at the door from where your head position is in the bed without turning your head. This is called the command position. However, never angle your bed so that your feet point directly toward the entry door. If your feet point toward the entry door, avoid this angle; it is called "the coffin position."

5. Mirrors in the bedroom are like having a third person present, and the additional reflection is not restful. Therefore, no mirrors in the bedroom.

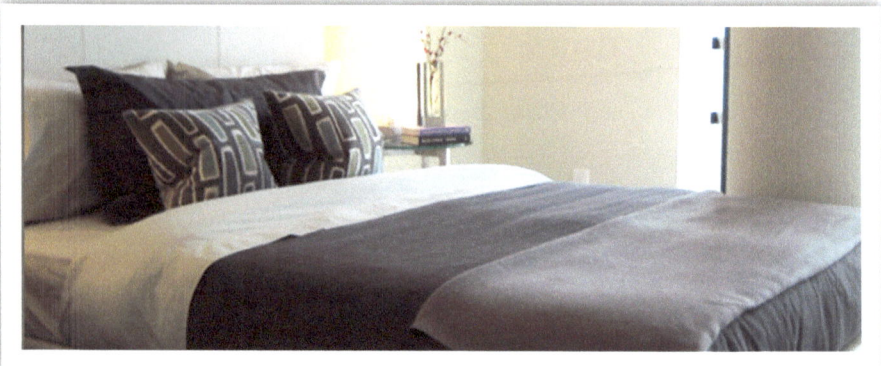

Photo Credit: Bethany St. Clair

6. Want to attract a partner? Leave empty space in your closet, dresser drawers and other bedroom storage so your new partner can have a place to put his/her things when he/she is manifested. If your closets and dressers are stuffed full, you are telling the Universe that you don't have room for a partner at this time.

7. Avoid hanging shoe racks or other storage racks on the backs of doors or doorknobs. This creates unnecessary clutter and chaos at the entry of a room, which feels heavy and unwelcome.

8. If you are lucky enough to have a fireplace in your bedroom, make sure it works and you use it. If the fireplace isn't used or doesn't work, you are missing out on all the wonderful warmth and energy the fire element provides.

9. Do keep your sheets and bedroom regularly cleaned and dust free. Wash bedding, liners, and mattress pads as frequently as you feel comfortable. I recommend washing sheets weekly, and linens and mattress pads twice a month. Buy the most expensive bedding you can afford. Good bedding will last longer and the difference when sleeping under a fine cotton sheet is amazing.

10. Use soothing, restful, colors in the bedroom: greens, blues, and earth tones work well, along with some purples and various shades of pink.

The Bathroom

The bathroom is one of the first rooms we enter as we begin our day and prepare to greet the world. How do you present yourself to the world? The bathroom is also one of the last rooms we attend before retiring for the evening. Why not honor this room as a beginning and completion to a day?

11. Paint your bathroom a soothing color: perhaps in earth tones, warm blues or even a soft pink, or warm lavender. Avoid greens and yellows in a bathroom as these are the least flattering colors for any skin tone.

12. Put personal items away after use. Nothing is more unsightly than a used hairbrush or personal toiletries left out in the open. If you don't have storage space or are renting, containerize personal items and repurpose some old end tables or cabinets by painting them with fun colors and use them for extra storage space.

13. Keep your bathroom sparkling clean! Create a regular routine for cleaning and keep your routine simple.

14. Keep the clothes hamper in a bedroom closet rather than taking up space in the bathroom.

15. Keep the waste basket in an under-the-sink cabinet and out of sight if possible. Do the same with the toilet bowl cleaner brush.

16. Bring in some plants that have round leaves and do well in humidity such as bamboo. This will add some positive chi (energy) to the bathroom.

17. Colorful accent pieces can be added to create a theme. For example, if you like the ocean, add some shells and colorful towels, or artwork with a shell motif.

18. If you're short on shelf space, you can add a wall rack for towels, or open shelving. If your shelving is open, use baskets as containers for personal items such as: make-up, body products, hygienic items, etc. The baskets will conceal these items.

19. Locate an extra long shower curtain and hang the rod (if you have an expandable one) higher toward the ceiling. The room will appear much larger.

20. The bathroom is not the library. Remove all books, magazines, etc. If you are sitting on the commode for too long, change your diet. Eat more fiber.

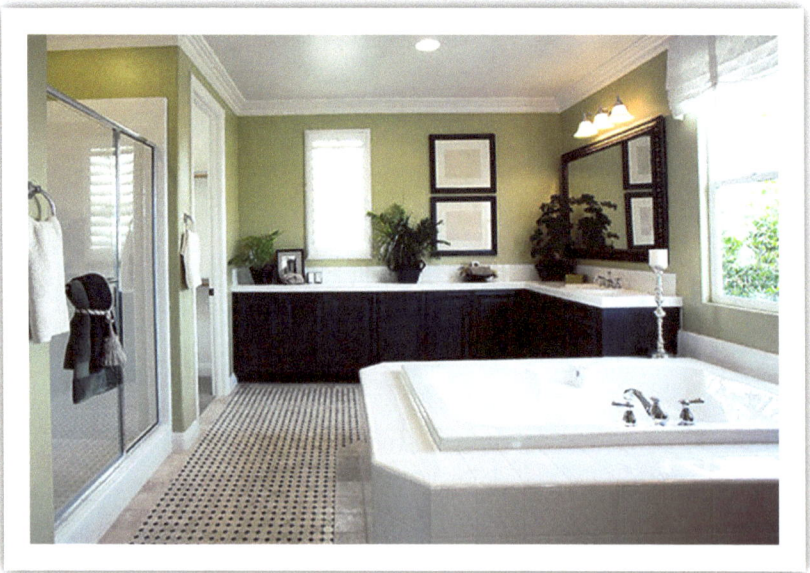

Photo Credit: Consumer Reports

The Kitchen

The kitchen is the hearth of the home. Along with "great rooms" today, this area is often the gathering space of a home, the heart of the home, and the source of our nourishment. Ask: how do I nourish myself?

Here are some key tips for using organization and feng shui for the kitchen.

21. Make certain everything is working in the kitchen: lights, appliances, fixtures, etc. In feng shui, broken items equal bad energy. Either get broken items fixed, toss them out, or replace them.

22. As in the bathroom, it is important to keep the kitchen immaculate. Clean areas after usage.

23. No matter how large or small your kitchen is, keep as much surface space available for preparation as possible. Do this by putting items away after you use them.

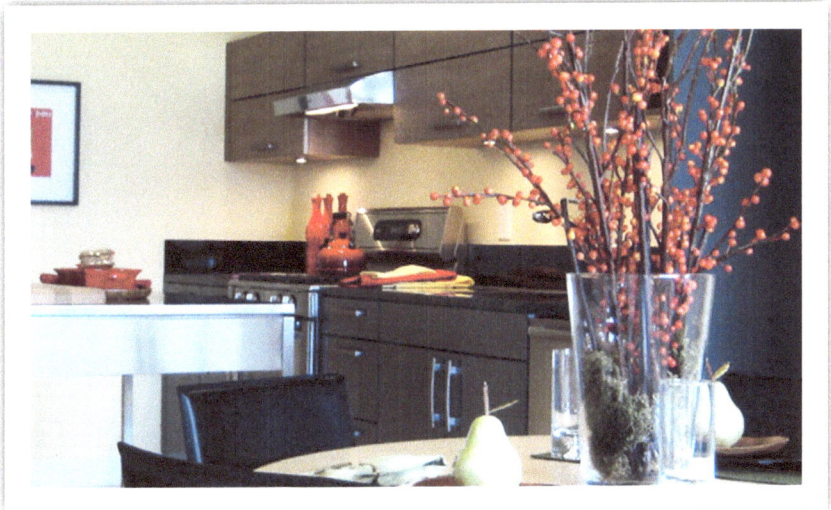

Photo Credit: Bethany St. Clair

24. Locate items near the zone that you use them. For example, the coffee supplies can go where the water source is, which would be near the coffee/espresso machine.

25. Items that you use every day can be kept in an easily retrievable location, I call this the "daily zones." Items that are seasonal can be kept in a space farther away from the daily zones.

26. Back-up supplies and large bulk items can be placed in the garage or pantry area. If you've ever worked in a restaurant, there is a storage space for back-up supplies. Regularly check these areas for inventory and purchase accordingly.

27. One of the ways to save money with groceries and supplies is to plan meals ahead of time and keep food storage spaces well-organized and stocked. Also, if you're in a multi-occupant living situation, assign tasks for who does the shopping, cleaning, preparing, etc. Then rotate the tasks weekly or monthly. It helps to have a responsibility sheet or assignment sheet as a checklist so each person will be clear on expectations, etc. One of the biggest ways I've seen families waste money is the double-purchasing of items. Know your inventory.

28. A great way to magnify your prosperity is to put something reflective on the backsplash area of your stove, such as a mirror.

29. If your kitchen doubles as an office zone, make sure your office supplies are in concealed containers. Label items and add shelving if necessary to keep office supplies in the office zone.

30. Each night before you go to bed, make sure the kitchen and the kitchen sink are cleaned and everything is put away. Wash the dishes before you go to bed and when you wake up in the morning, put the dishes away. It is very satisfying to wake up to a clean kitchen and helps you begin your day with clarity.

Children's Bedrooms

Like adults, children need their rest, and even more so. Back in my childhood, we would be sent to our room for punishment. The first time I did this with my younger son, his eyes lit up. No wonder--here was his television, computer games, DVD's, and guitar!

Children today have way too many play things in their bedroom, and parents often use children's rooms as a storage space for their own stuff. With the exception of a few night-time reading books and their favorite personal artwork, keep the children's rooms simple and clutter-free. One of the most important functions for a child is to get a good night's rest. The other is to eat nutritionally well. All the tips mentioned in the master bedroom apply to a child's bedroom.

31. Pay particular attention to the "zones" in your child's bedroom. By this I mean, how many areas in the room are dedicated to specific activities? There should be no more than three activities/zones in any room. For the bedroom, the obvious activity is sleeping. Another would be reading, and a third could be closet and dressing area. That's it.

32. Keep a child's bedroom restful by using pale colors and go brighter by adding a few accent colors.

33. Make sure your child has a good quality bed and mattress.

34. Open the windows and allow for fresh air in the bedroom. I can't tell you how many children's bedrooms are stuffy, have poor lighting, and poor air circulation.

35. If your living space is so small that you need to put toys and other items in the children's bedroom, make sure items are stored out of sight in manageable-sized containers and put away when not in use.

36. Children need to know where to put things. Give them a template to follow by creating zones and putting items at your child's height so they can easily retrieve and put things away. For example, locate clothing where items can be reached.

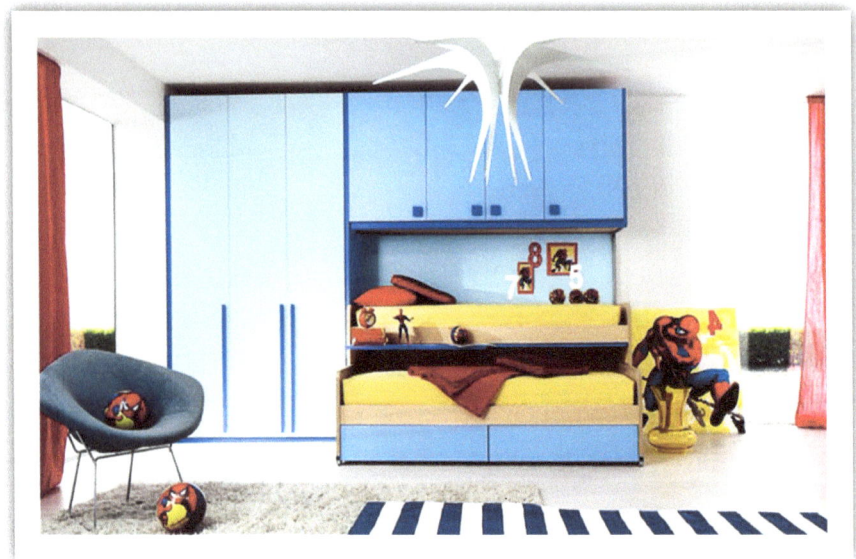

Photo Credit: ZG Group via Aldovega.com

37. It is helpful to establish a rewards system for doing various chores. Use a "star chart" and put this on your child's wall or post on the back of the closet door. Each night give your child a gold star when they have completed tasks. At the end of each week, give them a reward for their accomplishments. Be consistent!

38. Feng shui your love for your children. Ask yourself: do my eyes light up when my child walks into the room? Do I smile? If not, practice this!

39. Regularly purge your child's toys and clothing. Get your child involved and ask his/ her permission (yes, ask permission), to purge items that don't fit or aren't being used. Take your children with you to donate books, toys, or clothing so they can be knowledgeable of the recycling process. Conversely, show them how to take care of their things and how to repair broken items. Be the example by caring for your items as well.

40. Avoid a television, computer, or video games in the children's bedroom as they are not restful to sleeping.

The Media Room

If you are fortunate enough to have a media room, this is a terrific place to locate computers, printers, television, and other electronic equipment. The space can then be shared by other family members, which is good for parental oversight of minors.

As of this writing, media rooms are now frequently what used to be the family room. This is a very functional option for a growing family. When the children grow up, the room can be converted back to a family room. Below are some feng shui tips for the media room.

41. Have appropriate window treatment in the media room. These rooms become very warm from the use of electronic equipment, and having the right window treatment will keep the area fresh and well-lit.

42. Place some live plants in the media room. Plants provide oxygen for a space, and again with all of the EMF's floating around, plant life will balance the energy of the space.

43. Make sure there is good fresh air circulation in this room and dust frequently. Dusty rooms hold old energy and make a space feel heavy. If you find yourself yawning often, it is probably time to dust. Set up a schedule for dusting; both light dusting and heavy dusting.

44. Be sensitive to noise levels in the media room. Sound is energy. If more than one function and more than one person are in the room at the same time, consider using headphones so as not to disturb the other occupants.

45. One of the best ways to absorb excess sound is with the proper floor treatment. Manufactured hard floor treatments have a sharper sound, while natural wood flooring has a deeper sound. Low pile, industrial-type carpeting absorbs sound well in the media room, or area carpet/rug treatments work well also.

46. Check EMF levels in your home and particularly the media room. This can be done by purchasing an EMF detector or sensor. Many different brands can be found on the internet. As stated earlier, high levels of EMF's in your home or workplace can weaken the human immune system.

47. Keep food out of the media area. This is better for the digestive system and also less risk of a liquid spill on your computer.

48. If you're feeling tired from the EMF's or generally lethargic when doing a lot of computer work, wear a color that feels invigorating to you.

49. Think about what your functions for the media room are. How the space will be used most of the time? For example, if there will be a lot of computer work, studying, and homework in this room, consider painting the walls yellow. Yellow is a good color for clarity. If this will be a room where there is more television and movie watching, consider the color green, which is good for community, family life, grandparents. (See bonus feng shui tips at the end of this book).

50. If this is a family gathering place, then this is a great place to hang current family photos.

The Home Office / Your Work Office

If you are fortunate enough to have a separate room or space for your home office, this section is for you. Otherwise, all of these tips can be implemented at your workplace away from home.

51. Much like the master bedroom, make sure your desk is located in the "command position." (See master bedroom tips.) Too many times a desk will be located under a window facing out away from the entry of the room. The desk should be positioned at the opposite end of the room from the entryway, and so the occupant can see the entryway without turning.

52. Have some live plants in the office. Add a fountain for a water element, unless you live by the water; then no fountain is needed.

53. Side or desk lighting is preferable to overhead lighting. Overhead makes a space feel industrial (if you like an industrial look, then use overhead lighting). Side or desk lighting softens the space.

54. As you enter the home office, make sure that the focal point from the entry is the desk. Other items such as printers, etc. create a cluttered feel. If possible, place these on the wall at the same side as the entry, and if you do this, the office will look and feel less chaotic upon entering.

55. Sit at your desk in your office. What do you see? If you see clutter, then clean up the area you are looking at and replace items with a soothing visual. For example, a favorite piece of art, or an item that brings you joy, or even a plant or favorite chair. Now when you sit down at your desk, you are receiving joyful energy from items you love. Always surround yourself with items you love. Soon the work becomes enjoyable.

56. If you have miscellaneous items in your office that are not regularly used, put them in a cabinet with a door if possible. In this fashion, you can easily retrieve them when needed, but they won't be visible.

57. In an office space, think: location, location, location. By keeping the items you use the most closer to you, you will save time and be more efficient. For example, if your printer is within arms-reach, then keep the printer paper next to the printer.

58. When working on anything that takes three minutes or less to do, do it right then and check it off your list.

59. Studies have shown music by Mozart, or Baroque music stimulate the brain. Try playing this music in the background while working on a project.

60. Get to work ten minutes early every day! Getting to work early is a calmer way to set up your priorities for the day, and perhaps give you some individual face-time with your boss, who will notice your good habits.

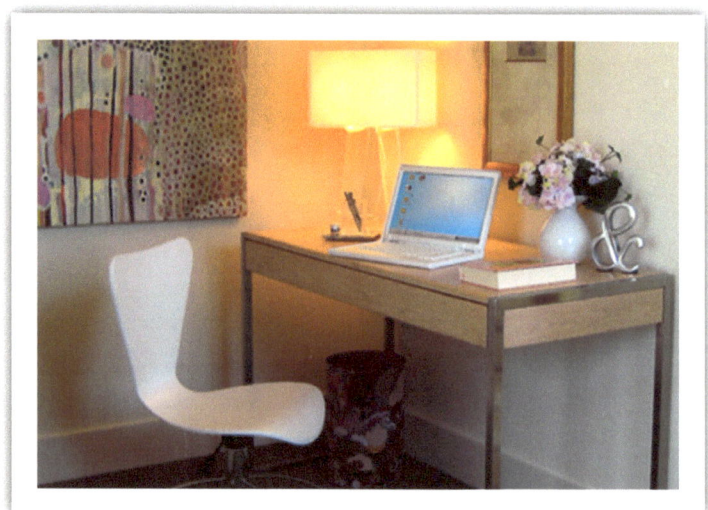

Photo Credit: Bethany St. Clair

The Great Room

The great room is featured more and more in homes and residences as part of our modern living. Great rooms are a gathering space. This is the one place that may have more than three zones because the great room is created for multiple activities. There will probably be an informal eating area, a food prep (kitchen) area, and a media area that doubles as an activity area. The key, as in all other areas of the home, is not to mix up the zones. When we keep the supplies of an activity in the correct zone, we tend to complete the things we started. For example, we may choose to use the dining room table to pay bills; the key is to put the bills and supplies away in a container after using them. Even more importantly, if we haven't created a process for the bill paying, then we will mix up the zones, and bills will get scattered in several different places. Below are some organizing and feng shui tips for the great room.

61. The great room is a perfect place to use containers for zones. If you have children, use a wicker basket for kids to drop their backpacks when they come home from school. Each child can have their own labeled basket.

62. Have pets? The pet should have his/her own zone as well: a pet bed for napping and sleeping, a zone for pet eating that should be away from human eating, and a zone for pet food that should be away from human food.

63. Adding extra cabinets in the great room is a useful way to create extra storage for supplies. For example, if you have craft supplies, put items in containers for the craft zone.

64. Pay attention to the noise and sound level in the great room. (See section on Media Room).

65. Gather your family or self at least one hour before you go to bed and pick up the great room, spend no more than thirty minutes on this task. By doing this, you'll have some buffer time from when you actually get ready for bed to when you hit the pillow. The reward is: when you wake up in the morning a clean, organized space welcomes you!

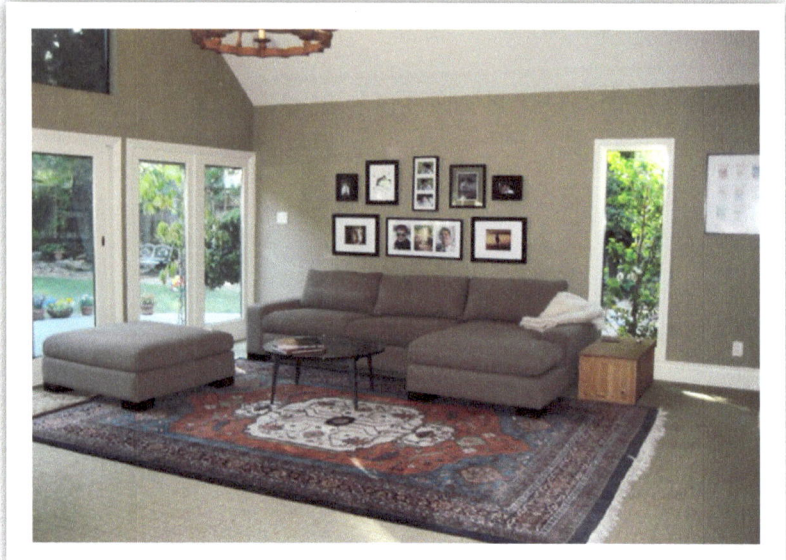

Photo Credit: Bethany St. Clair

66. Sweep or vacuum the floor every day or every other day. Energy from the day floats down from the space and collects there. The fresher your space is the fresher you'll feel.

67. The great room is a frequently used space. Keep the windows shiny clean. Open your arms and welcome yourself to the outside world.

68. Bring in fresh foliage or flowers from your outside space. Sometimes even the bushes have lovely branches that can be combined with florals or wildflowers. Using seasonal foliage is a lovely way to honor the cycles of nature.

69. Include fresh fruits and vegetables in your seasonal display. Again, this is a way to honor the outside world and the beautiful land we live in.

70. A great room is usually one of the largest rooms in the home. Make sure your artwork is scaled proportionally to the space. Many small items in a large space will look like clutter.
Use larger and fewer items to create more space and less clutter.

The Garage

The garage is one of the easiest spaces to organize. It is the area where energy gets stuck the most because it is filled with old items that are no longer useful or used.

Creating zones in the garage is the most effective way to create good flow. Think of the function of the garage: a space to hold your car! In many cases, our car is the second largest investment next to our mortgages. According to the Department of Transportation, 36% of cars are parked outdoors because there is no room in the garage.

Below are some tips for creating good flow in the garage.

71. Group like items together in zones. For example, keep holiday items together so seasonal retrieval will be easier. Have a zone for tools and workbenches. Have another zone for outdoor and sports gear.

72. Place frequently used items closer to the home entrance for quick retrieval, especially if the garage is attached to the home. For example, if you are fortunate enough to have space for back-up dry goods and pantry items, place those items close to the entrance of the home.

73. Containerize, containerize, containerize. Shelving, cabinets and plastic storage bins with snap lids are great products to help contain and retrieve items in their proper zone.

74. OPS - Other People's Stuff. If items in the garage belong to someone other than you, ask permission to move or touch their stuff. It is their inventory and you mostly likely wouldn't appreciate it if someone messed with your stuff without permission. Be respectful. If the owner says, "no," then let it go and focus on your stuff. Be a good role model. Better yet, organize with them and turn a lonesome task into a fun, group project. Reward the group when finished.

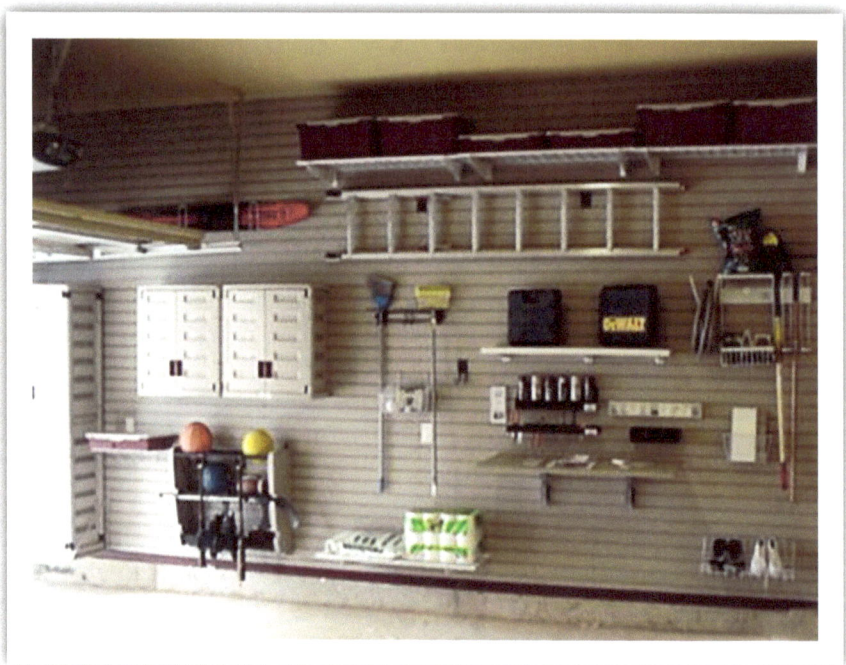

Photo Credit: HomeEdit.com

75. Establish a regular cleaning and organizing of the garage. Purge items that are no longer being used, unfinished, or outgrown. You may wish to schedule the garage for a quarterly, or twice-yearly purge.

76. There is a fortune sitting in your garage. Have a garage sale and get your neighbors involved. Even if you live in an apartment building, you can still have "sidewalk garage sales."

77. Consider safety issues in the garage, especially if you have small children. Keep toxic and poisonous items in their original containers, clearly marked and out of reach. For example, don't put toxic items in a Coke can where a child may think the contents contain a soft drink. Each year the Poison Control Center has heartbreaking stories of children who have died because of careless, preventable mistakes. The same goes for your beloved pets.

78. Design tip for painting the garage: paint the exterior of the garage door the same color as the body of the house, instead of "garage door white." This will make your home look larger and longer if the garage is attached to the house. If the garage is not attached to the house, do the same and the property will flow better.

79. If the roof of your garage has a "peak shape" above the garage door, consider putting a decorative item in this space to pull the eye upward instead of on the door. If you don't have a "peak shape," consider putting lanterns on either side of the garage door and make sure they match the outdoor light at the front door. When these lights are turned on at night, your home will look warm and cozy.

80. If you have a two-car garage, place an industrial carpet runner in-between the two cars so that when you exit the car, your feet will hit the runner and reduce the amount of dirt and grime you bring into the house.

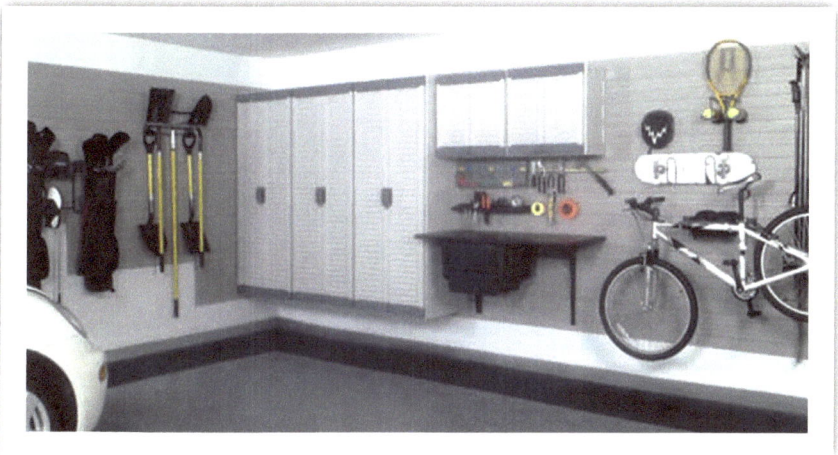

Photo Credit: LetsFixUpYourHouse.com

The Entryway

The entryway of your home is considered the "mouth of the chi" or the main energy point in your space. This is where all energy begins and sets the tone for your home and is the first impression your guests have of your space, so make the entryway feel welcoming.

Tips for the outside entryway:

81. Make sure the outside area of your front door is immaculate. Regularly clear out the cobwebs. Clean off the glass door and outside light. Make sure your outside and inside lights are always working. Daily, if not every other day, sweep the front porch area.

82. Paint your front door red or purple if this goes with your color scheme. These are powerful colors and magnify the energy of the entry point. If these colors don't work, go to the paint store and ask the specialist to suggest a complementary color.

83. Add live, colorful flowers to your entryway if possible but keep them simple. In other words, don't choke the entryway with plants. This will suffocate the energy from flowing in and cause chaos.

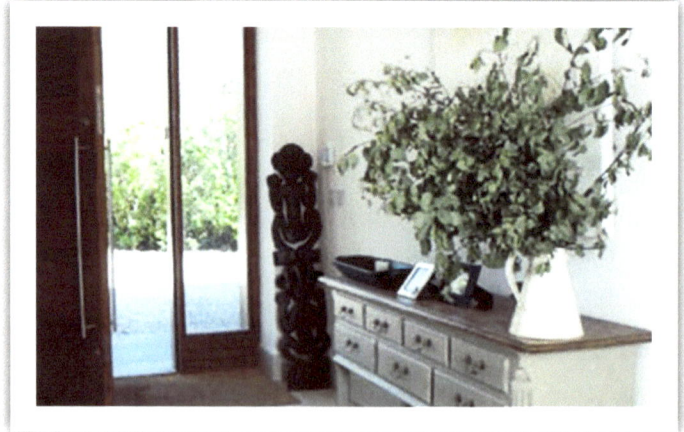

Photo Credit: NewStyleHouse.com

84. Keep the house numbers on the front of your house either in a horizontal position or a diagonal "upward" position. If on the diagonal, the first number on the left should be the lowest and the following numbers should be angled upward. In this fashion, the energy will feel "uplifted." Trust me; it works!

85. Make sure you use the front entryway. So many times we come into our homes from the garage and the entryway becomes an afterthought. Use it to keep the chi moving; otherwise, energy gets stuck.

Tips for the inside entryway:

86. The shoe thing: more and more, western homeowners are leaving shoes at the entryway, as is customary in the Orient. This is good because the energy from the grit and grime of urban or rural dwelling doesn't enter the home. However, the question becomes what to do with all the shoes? Consider built-ins at the entryway for shoes. Many furniture stores now carry cabinets and benches specifically made for shoes. Try and keep the shoes out of sight by putting them away in cabinets at the entryway.

87. If you ask guests and residents to take their shoes off at the entryway, be sure to provide slippers for them to put on. These can be arranged in a lovely basket at the entryway, similar to the manner in which we keep umbrellas in an umbrella stand.

88. Have a proportionally scaled area rug or runner at the entryway of your home. By doing this, the rug will ground the space, reduce noise, and set an inviting tone for the residence.

89. Make sure to have the inside entryway well lit. This creates a lovely, warm, inviting feel to your home or space, especially if the light comes from a table lamp vs. a harsh overhead light.

90. Add a happy piece of artwork at the entry, perhaps above a console table and a live plant. Again, the artwork, plant, and table, set the tone for the remainder of the space.

Closets

There is no reason why your closet can't look like a high-end department store. Everyday we get up and present ourself to the world. Unfortunately, most people judge us by the way we look, and until the world becomes a more altruistic place, this will continue. So for now, if we dress better we typically tend to get treated better.

Fact: we only wear twenty percent of what we own. The rest tends to sit there and collect dust. It would be easy to advise; get rid of the other eighty percent, but since we're creatures of habit, this is highly unlikely.

Clothing and what we wear clearly depends on our lifestyle, but know this: the more organized your closet is, the more time you'll have to enjoy the things you love to do rather than taking the time to find stuff. Below are some tips:

91. Set up your closet how you wear items on your body. The top shelf is for hats, scarves, then shirts and tops on the next rod, and on the lower rod are skirts, pants, and slacks. Have a separate space for long-hanging items, such as evening wear, dresses, etc. At the bottom of your closet should be footwear.

92. Whenever possible; use double-hanging rods to separate tops and bottoms. Double-hanging rods (one rod above and one below) provide double the space.

93. If you have a partner and must share a closet, create a side for you, and the other for your partner.

94. Hang classifications together and then sort by color, from light to dark. For example, hang long-sleeved shirts together, then sort by color. Next hang short-sleeved shirts together and then sort by color.

95. Sort footwear by season and classification: boots together, sneakers together, etc.

96. Delicate fabrics such as cashmere should be folded; otherwise they "grow" on the hanger.

97. Sort accessories by color and lay them flat.

98. Use fabric containers for undergarments and sort them separately; bras with bras, panties with panties, etc. This saves time putting items away after laundering and for easy retrieval when needed.

99. Use linen spray to freshen the smell of clothing. Spray far enough away so the clothing won't spot. Note: do not spray on fine fabrics such as silk.

100. Go through closets and drawers twice a year and edit your inventory. Donate or consign unwanted items.

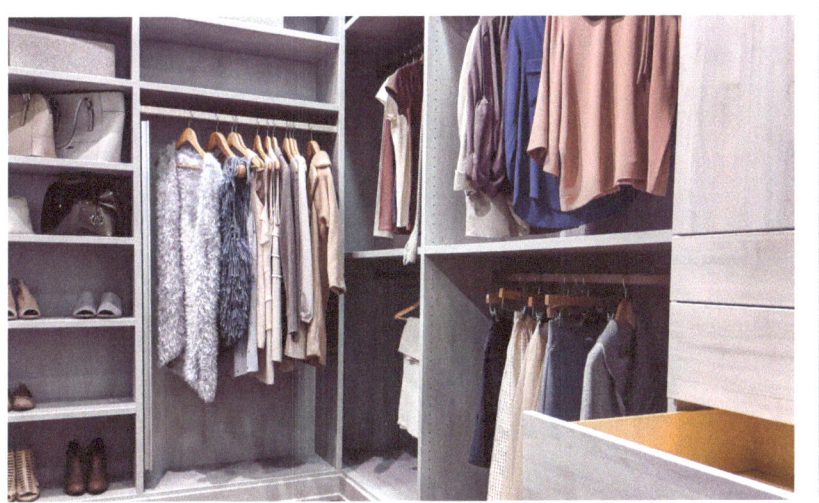

Photo Credit: Colleen Michaels/iStockphoto.com

Bonus Feng Shui Tips

The main rooms of the house are the focus in this ebook. Hence, the inclusion of other rooms such as: the basement, the dining room, music room, or guest room, study, etc. are omitted. However, below are some additional and repeated feng shui tips that can be used for any room in the house.

101. Keep the clutter under control. Clutter blocks energy and creates chaos. Remember, feng shui is the flow of things. Use the C-L-E-A-R process mentioned on my website (www.bethanystclair.com) for methods to reduce clutter.

102. Stuff on the floor pulls your heart energy down and can affect your moods. Keep clutter and even decorative items off the floor.

103. Make technology work for you. Old 8-track tapes, and cassette tapes are cumbersome and take up a lot of room and create dust. Let go of old technology and have fun learning about new technology. In the end, your life will be simpler.

104. If you have bookshelves and bookcases, keep each shelf 2/3 full. This way, you are making space for new information to come into your life.

105. Carefully look at your current artwork. Ladies, if you are trying to attract a man into your life, having pictures of single women or groups of women in your home will send messages to the Universe that you want to remain with your girlfriends. Instead hang pictures of couples.

106. If you have pictures of people toiling and you feel you are working too hard, change the pictures with artwork that reflects restfulness or fun. Your art should reflect what you desire in your life, what you value.

107. Everything, everything in your home or space holds en-ergy. Hence, the energy with our stuff is tied to our emotions. Surround yourself only with things you love. If you don't love it and you don't use it, let it go!

108. OPS = Other People's Stuff. Touching and moving OPS without permission is disrespectful. Always ask permission. If they refuse, let go of trying to control that person and focus on your own organization. Be a good role model. If you're still uncomfortable ask the other person if you can call in a professional organizer.

109. The front door or entryway is the "mouth of the chi." Make sure this space is immaculate, warm, inviting, and well lit. Remember, this is also how you'll be greeted when you return home. Your home should feel like you are getting a warm embrace every time you enter your space.

110. Careful consideration of sound in your home or workspace can have a profound affect on your mood and health. Sound carries energy. Pay attention to the sound in your space, especially when moving to a new location.

111. Use color to enhance the eight life areas of the ba gua. There are many types of feng shui, so select the type that resonates the most with you and study the ba gua.

Here are the basic colors for life enhancements when you stand at the entryway of each room, or look at a floor plan:

- Purple in the far left corner enhances prosperity, empowerment, wealth.
- Red in the far center location of a room enhances fame, future, luck.
- Pink in the far right area enhances relationships, partnerships, and marriage.
- White in the mid-right of a room enhances children, creativity, feminine energy.
- Grey in the near right area enhances helpful people, travel, masculine energy.
- Black in the near center area enhances life's journey, career, business success.
- Blue in the near left area enhances knowledge, wisdom, contemplation.
- Green in the mid-left area enhances community, family life, grandparents.
- Yellow in the center area of a room enhances health, unity, and well-being.

You can also use these colors and probably already do on a subconscious level when you dress. Some days you may feel like wearing purple, other days blue, etc. There is no right or wrong but by putting your attention on how colors relate to life areas will often create more awareness and sometimes humorous synchronicities in your life.

Once your space is clutter-free and your clearing systems are in place, you can then begin to go deeper with feng shui by studying furniture placement and using colors and articulating intentions to create the life you were born to live.

For additional information or to ask any questions, feel free to email me at info@bethanystclair.com. I look forward to your comments on this book.

www.ingramcontent.com/pod-product-compliance
Lightning Source LLC
Chambersburg PA
CBHW042054290426
44110CB00006B/180